GLUCOSAMINE SULFATE

and

CHONDROITIN SULFATE

by
Rita Elkins, M.A.

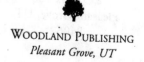

WOODLAND PUBLISHING
Pleasant Grove, UT

© 1997
Woodland Publishing
P.O. Box 160
Pleasant Grove, UT
84062

CONTENTS

GLUCOSAMINE SULFATE

An Overview

Glucosamine is a relatively new supplement which has some very exciting prospects as a natural and safe treatment for osteoarthritis and other inflammatory joint conditions. It offers an inexpensive and safe alternative to a whole host of arthritic drugs, and in many cases, can actually provide better relief that prescription or over-the-counter medications. Various studies have found that by adding glucosamine back to the body in supplement form, connective tissue healing and regeneration is enhanced. This particular action is invaluable for anyone suffering from diseases related to cartilage destruction. Of particular interest is the fact that glucosamine treats the root of osteoarthritis rather than just alleviating its symptoms as do standard drug therapies. In addition, unlike NSAIDs, it is considered very safe and non-toxic and can be used for extended periods of time without risk.

Unquestionably, anyone who suffers from osteoarthritis should acquaint themselves with glucosamine therapy. Of all the natural alternative treatments for arthritis, it may hold the most promise. Unfortunately, while some physicians are aware of the benefits of glucosamine, most are not. The clinical studies referred to in this booklet come from credible, academic sources and provide scientific documentation of the value of glucosamine for joint disease, especially in cases of osteoarthritis

What is Glucosamine Sulfate?

Glucosamine sulfate is a naturally occurring amino-monosaccharide found in highly concentrated amounts in the joints of mammals. When taken as a dietary supplement, glucosamine appears to be able to significantly restore normal biochemistry in supporting the rebuilding and healing of osteoarthritic cartilage. It is ideal as a supplement in that it supports cartilage function/repair over extended periods with no toxic side effects.

The body recognizes glucosamine as a natural substance, therefore it does not react to its presence in a negative way. It does not artificially suppress or stimulate normal cellular function, but rather augments physiological processes which have deteriorated with age, causing the gradual destruction of cartilage stores.

The Role of Naturally Occurring Glucosamine

The primary purpose of glucosamine is to stimulate the production of cartilage compounds and components which are necessary to keep the joint functioning and in a state of constant repair. The primary action of glucosamine in the human body is to prompt the production of connective tissue. Connective tissue comprises the fibrous material that binds our skeletal components together and is the main constituent of cartilage. Some body structures are totally made from connective tissue; notably, tendons and cartilage.

Connective tissue also forms the matrix (ground substance) of bone and the nonmuscular component of arteries and veins. Three primary types of cartilage exist and all are made up of special cells called chondrocytes which are embedded in the matrix. The matrix contains varying amounts of collagen, a gel-like substance. Hyaline cartilage is the tough smooth tissue which lines the surface of joints, such as the knee and provides an almost frictionless cushion over the bony regions of the joints. It is this lining that frequently wears thin with osteoarthritis, resulting in joint pain and restricted movement.

Glucosamine is actually the first biochemical component of connective tissue. In other words, it provides the body with the material required to manufacture the substance. It only stands to reason that replenishing the body with glucosamine would greatly enhance the synthesis or repair of new, much needed tissue in affected joints.

OSTEOARTHRITIS: A DEBILITATING DISEASE

Arthritis may be the oldest and most treated diseases in the history of mankind. For generations, tonics and potions with the promise of curing this debilitating disease have been created and readily sold. Arthritis is characterized by an inflammation of the joints with accompanying pain, swelling and stiffness. Osteoarthritis typically strikes older people, and is the most common form of arthritis. It affects over 80 percent of people over the age of fifty. Statistics indicate that over 40 million Americans suffer from some degree of osteoarthritis. Osteoarthritis is the leading cause of physical disability in the United States.

Typically it is our weight-bearing joints which are most affected by osteoarthritis as well as the joints of our hands. The course of the disease involves progressive cartilage destruction and hardening followed by the formation of bone spurs in joint cavities. Without the presence of healthy cartilage, our joints lose their "shock absorbers" making them vulnerable to wear and tear. When joint protection is compromised, joint and bone damage results with subsequent partial or complete immobilization and sometimes deformity. Something as seemingly innocuous as cartilage is what enables us to move freely and without pain.

Causes of Osteoarthritis

While rainy, damp weather does not cause arthritis, it definitely seems to aggravate the condition. Osteoarthritis may be caused by a number of age-related factors including an altered biochemistry which causes a decline in certain biocompounds and hormones. This condition typically attacks the knees, hips, and fingers and occurs when cartilage cushions which line the joints become stiffer and rougher. Consequently, bone can actually overgrow the joint area causing swelling and decreased movement. In its final stages, arthritic pain may actually subside; however, at this point, the joint has become totally immobile. Heredity may also play a factor is determining who is susceptible to developing osteoarthritis. The following list identifies many common causes of arthritis: age-related changes in collagen synthesis and repair, fractures or other trauma to bones or joints, genetic predisposition, altered biochemistry due to other diseases or foreign substances, hormonal dysfunction, excessive wear and tear, and inflammatory joint disorders

Symptoms of Osteoarthritis

In its initial stages, the symptoms of osteoarthritis can be very mild and hardly noticeable. Arthritis may be limited to only one joint or may affect many. Initially, one may notice that after a certain activity, a joint may feel sore. As the disease progresses pain, stiffness and limitation of use occur. Depending on the joints it affects, the symptoms of arthritis can vary somewhat.

The following symptoms are typically experienced during the course of osteoarthritis: morning stiffness, swelling, recurring tenderness in one or more joints, changes in ability to move joint, redness or feeling of warmth in joints, and in severe cases, deformity. Local tenderness, creaking and cracking of joints, edema and pain that worsens the more the joint is used are also signs of osteoarthritis. Morning stiffness is often the first symptom of the disease.

Standard Medical Treatment of Arthritis

NSAIDs are some of the most widely prescribed drugs in the United States, a fact which strongly suggests that pain has become a way of life for most Americans. Unfortunately, because of their accessibility and the free manner in which these drugs are prescribed, they are taken liberally for everything from a slight headache to severe arthritic pain.

Traditionally, aspirin was used to treat the pain and inflammation of arthritis. Aspirin, along with several other drugs belongs to a class of medications called NSAIDs (nonsteroidal, anti-inflammatory drugs). While aspirin may be effective in the initial stages of the disease, as the condition worsens, very large therapeutic doses are required which often create toxic side effects, including a ringing in the ears, gastrointestinal irritation and blood thinning.

Today, other NSAIDs are commonly prescribed by doctors for arthritis and include Ibuprofen (Advil, Nuprin, Motrin etc.), Indomethacin (Indocin, Indometh, Naprosyn), Fenoprofen (Nalfon) and Meclofenamate (Meclomen, Meclofen). While these types of NSAIDs may be better tolerated than aspirin, they are not necessarily more effective. In addition, they are quite costly and pose significant health risks when used over long periods of time and in certain dosages.

Using corticosteroids has also been a traditional treatment and poses even greater health risks. Steroid drugs should only be used as a last resort in cases where a physician has determined that it is absolutely necessary. Ironically, long-term use of steroid drugs can weaken bone structures and actually cause arthritic like conditions in some people.

Side Effects of NSAIDs

NSAIDs come with a whole host of undesirable side effects. In addition, prolonged use of this particular class of prescription and over-the-counter drugs may actually hasten the progression of arthritic disease. Certain studies have shown that NSAIDs inhibit the process of cartilage repair in that they impede the synthesis of collagen matrix.[1] Ironically, the disease mechanisms which cause osteoarthritis are actually boosted by the use of NSAID drugs. The fact that some studies strongly suggest that using these drugs may actually accelerate cartilage destruction is extremely significant and rarely addressed by medical practitioners. Most people who suffer from osteoarthritis are not aware of this particular undesirable action. Other side effects associated with NSAIDs include upset stomach, stomach ulcers, liver damage, kidney dysfunction, dizziness, tinnitus, lowered blood sugar, and abnormal heart rhythms. In addition taking Ibuprofen can increase the action of sulfa drugs, phenytoin, phenobarbital and anticoagulants. Anyone with kidney trouble, or who is pregnant or nursing should not take NSAIDs without their doctor's approval. Mixing alcohol with certain NSAIDs can be dangerous.

Millions of people take NSAIDs daily and thousands suffer with NSAID-related side effects. By contrast, glucosamine therapy offers a significant therapeutic benefit for arthritis sufferers without the deleterious side effects of NSAIDs and steroid drugs. Unfortunately, very few victims of rheumatoid disease are aware of the benefits and affordability of glucosamine treatment.

IS GLUCOSAMINE DEPLETION LINKED TO OSTEOARTHRITIS?

Recent studies on the profound role of hormone levels such as DHEA and HCG have strongly suggested that, to a certain degree, we age according to our diminishing supply of certain vital compounds. Time causes the cessation of certain hormones and the depletion of others causing a cascade effect which ultimately results in many of the geriatric debilities we are all acutely aware of.

One of these unfortunate events involves the ability to continually support healthy cellular growth. Regarding the condition of our cartilage stores, glucosamine stores play a profound role. When cellular regeneration is inhibited or impaired, many different ailments can result, including the development of osteoarthritis. Keeping our cartilage supple, flexible and in ample supply determine how well our joints function. Aging can cause cartilage to change, and in some ways become "petrified" or stone-like resulting in a lack of cushioning and subsequent degeneration. The glucosamine link to these physiological changes is what needs to be more thoroughly addressed.

Some scientists have theorized that when the body becomes unable to manufacture adequate supplies of glucosamine, susceptibility to developing osteoarthritis dramatically rises. Apparently, as we age, many of us lose the ability to produce the necessary levels of glucosamine we need to protect our joints. Consequently, the cartilage components of our skeletal frames lose their capacity to hold water, therefore, joint protection diminishes. The logical question here is: if the loss of glucosamine leads to arthritis, would restoring glucosamine slow the disease?

This notion prompted European clinicians and researchers to experiment with replenishing glucosamine supplies in people suffering from arthritis. The results were remarkable and somewhat unexpected. Several double-blind studies have demonstrated the fact the glucosamine sulfate may actually be superior to the use of NSAIDs (non-steroidal anti-inflammatory drugs) for the alleviation of arthritic pain and soreness.

Glucosamine Sulfate: A Non-Toxic Alternative to NSAIDs

Glucosamine is a non-toxic, natural substance which, unlike pharmaceutical drugs used to mask symptoms, treats the origin and cause of the disease. In other words, it acts more like a healing agent that a simple pain reliever. Not only does glucosamine provide some of the same benefits as anti-inflammatory drugs in controlling pain and inflammation, it actually contributes to the repair of joints which have deteriorated.

Compared with the significant health risks of taking NSAIDs, glucosamine is 10 to 30 times more desirable in its therapeutic action weighed against its safety.[2] A study conducted in 1992 concluded,

> In particular glucosamine sulfate, which naturally occurs in the human body and is almost devoid of toxicity is suitable for long-term therapeutic use . . .with its pharmacological rationale for the use of glucosamine sulfate as a disease-modifying agent in osteoarthritis.[3]

Another study published in 1991 concerning the safety and viability of glucosamine as a therapy for arthritis stated that "the pharmacological therapeutic index of glucosamine with regard to the anti-inflammatory activities seems therefore comparable or superior to that of the known non-steroidal anti-inflammatories."[4] Still yet another clinical study conducted with animal models concluded that "glucosamine sulfate can therefore be considered as a drug of choice for prolonged oral treatment of rheumatic disorders."[5]

A study published in January of 1994 concluded that oral applications of glucosamine sulfate were at least as effective if not more that non-steroidal anti-inflammatory drugs in relieving the symptoms which are commonly associated with arthritis. Using 155 patients with knee osteoarthritis, glucosamine was administered over a period of six weeks.[6] The remarkable results strongly suggested the use of glucosamine sulfate as a safer alternative to NSAIDs. "Glucosamine sulfate is a drug used in the treatment of osteoarthritis. When orally given, it is more effective than placebo and at least as effective as non-steroidal anti-inflammatory drugs in relieving osteoarthritis symptoms."[7]

Glucosamine vs. Ibuprofen

Clinical studies conducted in Portugal involving forty-eight patients who suffered from arthritis compared the action of Ibuprofen and glucosamine.[8] Test results revealed significant data differentiating between the action and mechanics of the two substances. Patients who took Ibuprofen drugs initially experienced quick pain relief over a period of two weeks. By contrast, the glucosamine users did not obtain as much pain relief over the same time interval. The testing continued and by the end of an eight week period the data took a flip flop. The Ibuprofen users were experiencing elevated pain levels while the glucosamine group was in significantly less pain.

What this study dramatically indicated was that time is an intrinsic part of glucosamine therapy and conclusions should not be drawn prematurely as to its effectiveness. As previously mentioned, we live in a society where we want immediate pain relief even if the analgesic may actually promote the disease process. Most natural treatments for disease involve more patience but can ultimately be more effective and even healing. The notion of a healing analgesic compound is rather foreign to modern-day pharmaceuticals. Obtaining relief while enhancing tissue repair is germane to the action of glucosamine.

Italian Studies on Glucosamine

Italian researchers conducted tests on the effects of glucosamine versus Indocin, a standard arthritic drug. Three groups of rats were used who had inflammatory conditions which mimic osteoarthritis or rheumatic conditions in human beings. While they found that Indocin was much more powerful than glucosamine in significantly lower amounts, they also discovered that its toxicity was 1000 to 4000 times greater than glucosamine.[9] Granted, the glucosamine was not as strong, but is was also considered completely safe and non-toxic. As a result of factoring in toxicity as a significant parameter of desirability, the Italian clinicians concluded that glucosamine sulfate should be considered the "therapy of choice" for the prolonged oral treatment of disorders like arthritis.

The anti-reactive activity of glucosamine sulfate . . . was tested on the rat in experimental models of subacute inflammation (sponge granuloma and croton oil granuloma), on subacute mechanical arthritis (kaolin arthritis) and in immunological-reactive arthritis and generalized inflammation (adjuvant arthritis). On these models, glucosamine was found effective in oral daily doses of 50-800 mg/kg.[10]

How Does Glucosamine Affect Arthritic Joints?

Ironically, with all the emphasis physicians place on using anti-inflammatory drugs to treat arthritis, glucosamine does not act as a direct anti-inflammatory. In other words, it does not initiate a direct pain-killing effect.[12] In this regard, glucosamine dramatically differs from the therapeutic action of NSAIDs, which are designed to only target arthritic symptoms and do not address the cause of the disease. While it does have anti-inflammatory properties, glucosamine acts to control inflammation in a completely different way than drugs like Ibuprofen. Unlike NSAIDs, glucosamine assists in the healing and regeneration of damaged tissue.

Glucosamine: A Disease Modifier, Not a Disease Masker

One of the most important differences between synthetic drugs and natural therapies is that in many cases, artificially synthesized chemical substances do little to promote healing, but rather address the notion of symptom management. While none of us would want to be without some of these very effective drugs, we must realize that because of their potency and origin, they come with significant side effects. Glucosamine is a natural compound that is easily assimilated and recognized by the body. Because it does not stress other organs, it can be used for an indefinite period of time without the fear of compromising one's health.

Osteoarthritis usually requires long-term therapy with NSAIDs or corticosteroids which do not repair damaged joints. Glucosamine, on the other hand, improves symptoms while boosting tissue regeneration, a feat that should not be underestimated. As is the case with most natural treatments, patience and persistence is the key.

Glucosamine: A True Chondoprotective Agent

The term "chondoprotective" refers to "cartilage" protective and certain medicinal agents which fall into this category were recently tested for their action and effectiveness in a study published in 1992. The results were fascinating and once again, reiterate the very unique mechanism of glucosamine sulfate, setting it apart from other so-called chondoprotective substances. Consider the following quote:

> The medicinal therapy of osteoarthritis is based on the use of analgesics, NSAIDs and corticosteroids to relieve pain and inflammation. In addition, "chondoprotective" agents (CPA) are used to stop the evolution of the disease. In this review the biochemical and pharmacological activities of some of the most widely used CPAs are described. All of these show more or less marked anti-inflammatory activities, which for some of them are the result of an inhibition of cyclo-oxygenase and of prostaglandin biosynthesis, in which case they should be more properly classified as mild NSAIDs. Only two of the CPAs reviewed, diacerein and D-glucosamine sulfate elicit anti-inflammatory and antireactive effects without significant inhibition of the prostaglandin biosynthesis. These agents have also remarkable chondoprotective effects, and only these two agents should be classified as true CPAs. In particular, glucosamine sulfate, which naturally occurs in the human body and is almost devoid of toxicity, is suitable for long-term therapeutic use. This with its chondometabo-like antireactive and antiarthritic properties, represent the pharmacological rational for the use of glucosamine sulfate as a disease-modifying agent in osteoarthritis.[13]

Glucosamine's Antireactive Properties

In a study published in February of 1991, glucosamine was tested for its anti-inflammatory activities and it "showed to protect against the edema provoked in the rat paw by carrageenin, dextran, formalin. . . . Furthermore glucosamine protected against peritonitis provoked in the rat by formalin and in the mouse by acetic acid."[14] While glucosamine did not inhibit every kind of irritation caused by different inflammatory agents, its performance was impressive enough to prompt the conclusion that it was the safest treatment of choice with an notable absence of toxicity in the gastrointestinal tract, a feature which eludes even the most sophisticated NSAID drug.[15] Ironically, NSAIDs pose their most significant threat to the lining of the gastrointestinal tract.

Glucosamine and HIV

Interestingly, in studying the physiological properties of glucosamine, one study found that it possessed significant anti-HIV-1 activity.[16] Currently, additional studies on the chemical properties of glucosamine are underway and are exploring its effect on various physiological functions.

Why Glucosamine is so Effective in Oral Supplement Form

While many other cartilage enhancing compounds are recommended for the treatment of arthritis, glucosamine is thought by many to be superior in its biochemical absorbability. Glucosamine is readily assimilated and absorbed while cartilage extracts, and chondroitin sulfate products are comprised of much larger molecules. Studies have found that up to 98 percent of orally administered glucosamine sulfate is absorbed in its entirety.[17] "After oral administration a proportion close to 90 percent of glucosamine sulfate is absorbed."[18]

After it is orally ingested, glucosamine is selectively taken up by cartilage structures where it initiates and boosts the production of much needed mucopolysaccharides. The liver eventually metabolizes a significant amount of glucosamine into smaller molecules and ultimately to CO_2, water, and urea. The ability of glucosamine to be so effective even when taken orally, makes it an ideal arthritic medicine. It is easy to take and goes directly to the source of the problem.

Safety of Glucosamine Therapy

Glucosamine sulfate is considered nontoxic, is easily tolerated and absorbed, and has no contraindications or adverse reactions. It does not interfere with the action of any other drugs and can be taken over long periods of time. Rare side effects include nausea or stomach upset. Taking glucosamine with meals helps prevent this.

Glucosamine Usage

In order to obtain optimal therapeutic results with glucosamine, long term therapy is suggested. Taking glucosamine orally has proven to be effective. It is important to keep in mind that, unlike the quick action of NSAIDs, glucosamine will take longer to produce desired results. Ironically, because so many of us want pain remedies that work immediately even if they don't heal, natural substances, herbs, etc. have often been shelved for more potent synthetic pharmaceutical drugs. The fact that most arthritis treatments involve long-term therapies further supports the use of glucosamine due to its non-toxicity. Glucosamine works with the body to treat arthritis directly rather than to only alleviate its symptoms.

Once glucosamine takes hold and its therapeutic effects become established, it should provide a superior source of treatment, even when compared to powerful doses of medications like Ibuprofen. Typically glucosamine is taken three times with meals a day at a dosage that should be determined by your health practitioner.

Availability of Glucosamine

Glucosamine sulfate supplements should be readily available in health food stores. It is important to differentiate between glucosamine sulfate and glucosamine hydrochloride. Capsulized glucosamine is the most common form of the supplement and should be purchased from reliable sources.

CHONDROITIN: THE PERFECT COMPLEMENT TO GLUCOSAMINE

Combining glucosamine sulfate with chondroitin sulfate has been remarkably effective in treating osteoarthritis in several animal and human studies. More and more research points to the effectiveness of this duo, which has been used as a safe and effective arthritis treatment in Europe. Glucosamine and chondroitin work together synergistically to initiate the production of new cartilage while protecting existing cartilage tissue. Unlike corticosteroid or NSAID treatments, this natural compound couple goes to the heart of the problem—treating the disease at its source rather than just masking the symptoms. Healing is the key word here. Anti-inflammatory agents do not heal or stimulate regeneration. They are designed to relieve pain and inflammation and are often ineffective. Both glucosamine and chondroitin are chondroprotective agents; an impressive attribute which does not describe current pharmaceutical drugs designed to treat the symptoms of osteoarthritis.

Data concerning treatment for osteoarthritis with both of these compounds is compelling to say the least. What one fails to accomplish, the other achieves. For example, glucosamine stimulates the production of cartilage, provides joint lubrication and helps to reduce pain and inflammation. Chondroitin complements glucosamine as it boosts cartilage synthesis, inhibits the enzymes which destroy cartilage molecules, promotes cellular nourishment and contributes to joint protection. The combined effects of glucosamine and chondroitin could be the single most effective answer for the many thousands who suffer from osteoarthritis.

A Technical Definition of Chondroitin

Chondroitin is a chemical compound comprised of a long chain of sugars. It is a natural compound found in some dietary sources such as certain animal tissues. Dietary chondroitin will usually become assimilated in various body cells such as cartilage tissue. The long chemical chains of chondroitin react with the spine of proteoglycan molecules located in cartilage areas of our joints. This reaction forms spaces within cartilage allowing for much better water retention and protection. By facilitating the creation of watery spaces in affected joints, chondroitin supports the cartilage mending action of glucosamine. These water cushions help to protect cartilage from deterioration and promote joint flexibility and motion. Like glucosamine, chondroitin works at the cellular level to alleviate what causes arthritis pain in the first place, a task which no existing prescription drug can accomplish.

What Does Chondroitin Do For Arthritic Joints?

The chemical structure of chondroitin helps to create a watery, shock-absorbing space within cartilage tissue. In other words, chondroitin helps to enhance the fluid protection within joint systems resulting in better lubrication and nutrient transport. When fluid can accumulate in this manner, cartilage which is usually destroyed by arthritic disease stays more flexible and exhibits greater strength. Chondroitin has the unique ability to draw in and retain the watery fluid which cushions our joints and makes them mobile. In addition, chondroitin appears to be able to inhibit the action of specific enzymes which breakdown cartilage tissue, contributing to its destruction. Apparently, other enzymes also exist which can prevent the proper transport of vital nutrients to cartilage tissue. Chondroitin interferes with them as well, giving cartilage the opportunity to stay intact and well-nourished. Moreover, chondroitin can stimulate the synthesis of proteoglycans, collagen and other cartilage molecules which contribute to the production of new cartilage cells.

In short the three most important actions of chondroitin sulfate are 1) it serves to protect existing cartilage from further destruction or premature damage, 2) it stimulates the synthesis of new cartilage, and 3) it facilitates the creation and retention of fluid cavities which serve to cushion joints.

Studies on Chondroitin

Various clinical tests support the efficacy of chondroitin therapy. Injections of chondroitin in patients suffering from severe osteoarthritis have resulted in excellent improvement in both pain and mobility. Italian researchers conducted a double-blind study with arthritic patients using chondroitin and a placebo. They found that even with a reduced amount of NSAID drugs, those individuals taking chondroitin continued to improve and their pain decreased. French studies using oral chondroitin supplements found that cartilage repair was significantly enhanced in those patients using a three month protocol of chondroitin. A Neapolitan study found that using 1200 milligrams of oral chondroitin resulted in considerable improvement with no side effects in patients who had marked osteoarthritic symptoms. Study after study has confirmed that chondroitin sulfate has the ability to stimulate cartilage repair, decrease joint pain and enhance mobility.

Why Don't Doctors Use Glucosamine and Chondroitin?

Unfortunately, once certain medical protocols are in place, attitudes and acceptance concerning unpatentable, natural treatments are rather ambivalent. The fact remains that both of these compounds have been proven safe and effective therapies for osteoarthritis. Because pharmaceutical companies cannot tout them as patented medicines to their pool of physicians, investing money in their promotion is simply not done. In the meantime, thousands of people suffer from arthritic pain and degeneration and have to suffer with ineffective or potentially dangerous anti-inflammatory drug treatments which do absolutely nothing to heal the cause of their disease. Amidst this medical anarchy, there is some cause for hope. More and more physicians are investigating natural therapies and their potential value. Compounds like glucosamine and chondroitin for osteoarthritis will not be ignored forever. Their impressive medicinal properties demand that they be further investigated. Moreover, data concerning their effectiveness gives them credibility among the scientific community.

Chondroitin and Glucosamine as Preventive Therapy

A physician who has recently written the best selling book, The Arthritis Cure, Jason Theodosakis, M.D., recommends using both glucosamine and chondroitin to lower one's risk of developing osteoarthritis. If this condition runs in your family, it may be prudent to take these two supplements on a daily basis. The apparent safety of both compounds suggests that these supplements may be taken over long periods of time. (NOTE: At this writing, scientists are attempting to improve substances which work like chondroitin to regenerate or replace damaged cartilage. The consensus is that in the near future, arthritis treatments will take a completely new direction—moving away from NSAIDS toward substances which heal, protect and regenerate joint cartilage.)

Safety Issues

Chondroitin sulfate is considered a nontoxic compound and using it over extended periods of time has resulted in no appreciable side effects.

Product Availability

Like glucosamine, chondroitin can be purchased in health food stores and some pharmacies. Forms of chondroitin include chondroitin sulfate and mucopolysaccharides. Make sure to buy pharmaceutical grade chondroitin to ensure purity and potency. It is not common to find both glucosamine sulfate and chondroitin sulfate in the same formula due to the fact that, until recently, glucosamine sulfate alone has been the more common treatment for osteoarthritis. As more data is compiled, products offering the two compounds in combination will undoubtedly emerge. At this writing using separate dosages of the two supplements is recommended.

Dosages

In order to receive the optimal therapeutic effect from chondroitin and glucosamine, adequate amounts of these compounds must be taken. According to Dr. Jason Theodosakis, the best way to asses how much to take is based on body weight. If you weigh less than 120 pounds, you need 1000 mg of glucosamine and 800 mg of chondroitin. Individuals between 120 and 200 pounds requires 1500 mg of glucosamine and 1200 mg of chondroitin. Those weighing more than 200 pounds need 2000 mg of glucosamine and 1600 mg of chondroitin. Dr. Theodosakis recommends that dosages should be adjusted according to results and advises that they be taken in two to four doses spread out over the course of a day. These supplements can be taken with or without food. (NOTE: Taking vitamin C, manganese, marine lipids and DHEA may help to enhance the effectiveness of a glucosamine/chondroitin protocol.)

Halting and Healing Arthritis

Anyone who is considering glucosamine therapy for osteoarthritis should add chondroitin sulfate to their therapeutic regimen. As of this writing, chondroitin is the most impressive cartilage regenerating substance available and should be implemented in natural treatment therapies for arthritic joints. Keep in mind that the progression of osteoarthritis involves faulty cartilage production and repair. Both proteoglycans and collagen synthesis decrease with age and as a result, many of us suffer from joint degeneration. The notion that natural and safe supplements not only prevent cartilage destruction, but actually contribute to its replenishment is remarkable, to say the very least. Glucosamine and chondroitin have the distinct ability to halt and heal the deteriorating processes caused by osteoarthritic disease without causing the severe stomach upsets created by continual NSAID use.

Both of these natural compounds work to repair cartilage damage that results from wear and tear or from disease processes. Together they form a new approach to treating joint diseases which epitomizes the difference between the holistic approach to disease and conventional treatments. Very few pharmaceutical preparations have the ability to actually heal. Keep in mind that just because various natural supplements are not sanctioned by the medical establishment or manufactured by powerful drug companies, they can still be of enormous value to the consumer. As more and more attention becomes directed at safer, more effective forms of disease treatments, natural compounds like glucosamine and chondroitin will emerge as viable therapeutic agents. It is only a matter of time. For more information on chondroitin, consult the following sources: Jason Theodosakis, M.D. M.S. M.P.H., Brenda Adderly M.H.A. and Barry Fox, Ph.D., *The Arthritis Cure.* (New York: St. Martin's Press, 1997); V. R. Pipitone, "Chondroprotection with Chondroitin Sulfate," *Drugs in Experimental and Clinical Research,* 17 (1), 1991, 3-7.

BIO-ENHANCING AGENTS

Ideally, glucosamine should be a part of a nutritional regimen designed to boost its overall effectiveness. A complete natural approach to osteoarthritis is preferable and addresses several factors which contribute to joint damage. Anytime the body is faced with a healing crisis, nutrition must be considered as a major player in promoting tissue repair and preventing further destruction. In addition, certain herbals and other substances can augment nutrition and enhance overall health and wellness. Specific vitamins, herbs and other constituents specifically complement glucosamine and speed healing.

Vitamins

Vitamin C with bioflavonoids: Because Vitamin C plays such an integral role in collagen synthesis and connective tissue regeneration it is crucial to any regimen designed to treat arthritic conditions. Clinical studies have established the value of Vitamin C for cartilage repair.[20] Interestingly, Vitamin C and E work in tandem to enhance the structure of vital cartilage constituents and are thought to prevent or minimize the deterioration of cartilage.

Vitamin E: Some studies have found that Vitamin E can also benefit people suffering from osteoarthritis.[21] Vitamin E has proven antioxidant actions and actually works to inhibit the breakdown of enzymes found in cartilage as well as enhance cartilage regeneration.[22]

Vitamin B3: Vitamin B3 also known as niacin can help to boost blood flow to affected joints by dilating small arteries. A complete array of all the B-vitamins is recommended in order to promote better balance and performance in the body.

Herbs

Devil's Claw: Devil's Claw (Harpagophytom procumbens) is a botanical which is indigenous to regions of Africa. It has quite a lengthy record of use for arthritis and has recently come under scientific scrutiny. Clinical studies involving animal models have found that Devil's Claw possesses an anti-inflammatory action that rivals phenylbutazone, a powerful synthetic drug.[23] Devil's Claw is more effective for the treatment of osteoarthritis than for rheumatoid arthritis. (Note: Some studies exist which dispute the anti-inflammatory action of Devil's Claw. It would only stand to reason, however, that if native Africans used this botanical as a traditional treatment for arthritis, the usage must have its basis in effectual therapeutic mechanisms.)

Cat's Claw: For generations, Peruvians have trusted in the anti-inflammatory attributes of Cat's Claw. Historically, it has ben used for arthritic joint conditions. Clinical studies conducted on the plant metabolites of Cat's Claw have discovered that it does inhibit the inflammatory response. The plant sterols found in Cat's Claw exhibited the ability to reduce artificially induced swelling in the paws of rats.[24] In addition, Cat's Claw also contains a source of proanthocyanidin, a phytochemical which acts as a potent antioxidant.[25] Because proanthocyanidins (sometimes referred to as pycnogenol) scavenge free radicals so effectively, they have shown some remarkable curative effects. Regarding arthritis, proanthocyanidins have proven their ability to significantly reduce joint inflammation.

Yucca: Yucca extracts have been successfully used as part of an arthritis protocol at the Desert Arthritis Clinic.[26] Some health practitioners consider yucca as a natural precursor to synthetic cortisone, which makes it useful in controlling swelling and inflammation.

Boswellia serrata: Modern medicine and pharmacology are just beginning to realize the value of this ancient natural substance. A gum resin which is harvested from large trees native to India, Boswellia has significant anti-arthritic properties. This gum resin also referred to as salai guggul and contains an acid which has shown its ability to control arthritis in a number of animal studies. Among its actions are the ability to inhibit inflammation through interfering with inflammatory mediators, improve circulation to affected joint tissues, and prevent a drop in glycosaminoglycan levels.[27] These studies strongly point to this interesting resin as a potentially viable treatment for both osteo-and rheumatoid arthritis.[28] No side effects or contraindications have been reported with Boswellia serrata.

Green Barley Juice: Green drinks made from green barley contain a whole array of nutrients including superoxide dismutase which helps to destroy the free radicals that damage the synovial fluid needed to provide adequate joint lubrication.

White Willow (Salix alba): This natural substance is extracted from white willow bark and is rich in salicylates, which are natural anti-inflammatory agents which help to ease the swelling and redness and are useful for joint and muscle pain.

Capsaicin Ointments: Clinical tests have confirmed that topical capsaicin ointments made from cayenne pepper can substantially alleviate the miserable pain that characterizes osteoarthritis and rheumatoid arthritis.[29] Ester Lipstein-Kresch, M.D. has studied the effectiveness of capsaicin creams for arthritis and has stated: "You need to apply it three or four times a day on the affected areas for at least two weeks before seeing any improvement. An initial burning sensation at the site is not unusual for the first few days, but this goes away with continued application."[30]

Garlic: Like proanthocyanidins, garlic helps to inhibit the formation of free radicals which can cause further damage to vulnerable joints. It also helps to boost cardiovascular health thereby enhancing better circulation to arthritic joints.

Other Nutritional Compounds

Shark Cartilage: Cartilage extracts can be found from both bovine and shark sources. Shark cartilage contains certain compounds known as mucopolysaccharides or glycosaminoglycans. One of the constituents of these molecules is called chondroitin sulfate which is actually comprises of chemical units of glucosamine sulfate combined with sugar. Dr. Jose Orcasita, M.D., tested the effectiveness of shark cartilage on several people suffering from arthritis and found that they experienced significant improvement.[31]

Subsequent studies conducted at the University of Miami School of Medicine found that arthritic pain could be substantially decreases by using shark cartilage extract. Dr. Orcasita stressed that fact that patients who took shark cartilage for arthritis experienced no side effects or toxicity of any kind. Apparently shark cartilage targets arthritis in two ways: first it acts as a natural anti-inflammatory to ease joint pain, and secondly, it helps to prevent the growth of an abnormal network of blood vessels that can develop in inflamed areas. The presence of these vessels significantly contributes to the pain and stiffness associated with arthritis. In 1988, Dr. Serge Orloff, a prominent European arthritis specialist obtained similar results in his studies. Some Eastern European data indicated that: arthritic pain could be decreased by 50 percent or more; a marked improvement in the quality of life was observed; increased function and activity resulted; and bedridden patients became ambulatory.[32] (Note: While the data on shark cartilage is promising, it should ideally be combined with glucosamine sulfate because glucosamine is much more absorbable. The chondroitin sulfate molecular content of shark cartilage in 200 times larger than glucosamine sulfate.[32] For oral consumption, the type of absorbability found in glucosamine is remarkable.)

Boron: Supplements of Boron have been utilized in Germany as a treatment of osteoarthritis for over three decades. A recent double-blind study evaluated its effectiveness and found that of patients who took 6 milligrams of boron, 71 percent experienced improvement as opposed to a 10 percent improvement rate seen in the placebo group.[33]

Methionine: This amino acid has proven its ability to rival the therapeutic effects of Ibuprofen in treating the pain typically present in cases of osteoarthritis.[34] The sulphur content of this amino acid is thought to support cartilage constituents including protoglycans and glycosaminoglycans.

Omega-3 Oils (fish oils or primrose oil): These oils contain Omega-3 fatty acids which provide substantial amounts of vitamin D, necessary for proper bone growth and function. It is also thought that fish oils compete with certain fatty acids that are believed to trigger arthritis inflammation in cases that are not age-related. These oils are also high in vitamin A, which may act as a natural anti-inflammatory.

Calcium and Magnesium Citrate: This very absorbable form of calcium and magnesium helps to fortify bones and works to prevent the bone loss that can sometimes result from advanced cases of osteoarthritis.

Proanthocyanidins (Pycnogenol): For joint injuries and arthritic conditions, proanthocyanidins (pycnogenol) which are extracted from grape seed or pine bark act as powerful anti-inflammatory compounds without any of the negative side effects associated with over-the-counter or prescription drugs. Proanthocyanidins bind with collagen fibers and help to alleviate arthritic pain and swelling.

They are considered much more powerful in their antioxidant action than vitamin C and E.

Foods Beneficial for Relieving Arthritis

Foods rich in bioflavonoids are recommended and include: blueberries, blackberries and cherries. In addition eat plenty of high fiber whole grains. Phytochemicals such as sulfur are also good and can be found in: onions, garlic, cabbage and Brussels spouts. Fresh raw fruits and vegetables contain live enzymes and are recommended, with the exception of those belonging to the night-shade family listed in the next section. All legumes including lentils, split peas and beans are good as well as fish and most seafood. (Note: Some studies have found a link between low sulphur content and arthritis.[35] Supplementing the body with doses of sulphur has been successful in some cases of arthritis for pain and swelling.[36] What these studies suggest is that eating a sulphur-rich diet and using sulphur supplements may be of great benefit for people with arthritis. Interestingly, glucosamine sulfate naturally contains sulphur compounds.)

Foods to Avoid

Arthritis sufferers should avoid fatty red meats, sugary rich foods, dairy products, egg yolks, soda pop, saturated fats, and in the opinion of some experts, vegetables considered part of the night-shade family which include: potatoes, peppers, tomatoes and eggplant. Dried fruits and salted nuts should also be avoided, as should nicotine and tobacco.

CONCLUSION

More and more people are turning to natural alternatives for the treatment of diseases like arthritis. Unfortunately, most of us exclusively rely on pharmaceutical agents which are continually touted to our corps of physicians as the latest and best treatments for specific diseases. While many of these drugs are useful, just as many natural therapies exist which work with rather than against the body's natural mechanisms to control pain and more importantly, promote healing.

Glucosamine sulfate is just such a compound and is relatively inexpensive and remarkably safe. It, more so than any other single natural therapy, holds the most potential for arthritis relief. Glucosamine treatment should be investigated and utilized by those of us who suffer from debilitating joint diseases. So often, the natural approach to treating disease can provide a better kind of pain relief without compromising overall health or endangering other body systems as do potent pharmaceutical agents.

As is the case with most natural substances, one must not expect to see overnight results with glucosamine. Patience and consistency are the key with this approach, which will unfortunately eliminate a number of people who may abandon the therapy before it has the chance to administer its beneficial effects. Clinical studies on glucosamine are clear and to the point—anyone who has osteoarthritis has everything to gain and nothing to lose by using glucosamine sulfate.

ENDNOTES

1 M.N. Newman and R.S.M. Ling, "Acetabular bone destruction related to non-steroidal anti-inflammatory drugs." LANCET. II: 1985, 11. See also P.M. Brooks, et al., 'NSAID and osteoarthritis, help or hindrance." JOURNAL OF RHEUMATOLOGY. (9), 1982, 3-5.

2 I. Setnikar et al., "Antiarthiric effects of glucosamine sulfate studied in animal models." ARNEIM-FORSCH. (41), 1991, 542-45.

3 I. Setnikar, "Antireactive Properties of 'chondoprotective' drugs." INT-J-TISSUE-REACT. 14 (5), 1992, 253-61.

4 I. Setnikar et al., "Antireactive properties of glucosamine sulfate." ARZNEIM-FORSCH. 41 (2), Feb. 1991, 157-61.

5 Setnikar, "Antiarthritic effects of glucosamine sulfate studied in animal models." 542-45.

6 A. Reichelt et al., "Efficacy and safety of intramuscular glucosamine sulfate in osteoarthritis of the knee: A randomized, placebo-controlled, double-blind study." ARNEIM-FORSCH. 44 (1), Jan. 1994, 75-80.

7 Ibid.

8 A. L. Vaz. "Double-blind clinical evaluation of the reactive efficacy of ibuprofen and glucosamine sulfate in the management of osteoarthrosis of the knee in out-patient. CURRENT MEDICAL RESEARCH OPINIONS. (8), 1982, 1450-59. See also G. Crolle and E. D'este, "Glucosamine sulfate for the management of arthrosis: A controlled clinical investigation." CURRENT MEDICAL RESEARCH OPINIONS. (7), 1981, 104-14.

9 Setnikar, "Antiarthritic effects of glucosamine sulfate studied in animal models." 542-45.

10 Ibid.

11 Ibid.

12 See Vaz, Setnikar, "Antiarthritic effects of glucosamine sulfate studied in animal models and Crolle.

13 Setnikar, "Antireactive properties of 'chondoprotective' drugs." 253-61.

14 Setnikar, "Antireactive properties of glucosamine sulfate." 157-61.

15 Ibid.

16 O. Bagasra, et al., "Anti-human immunodeficiency virus type 1 of sulfated monosaccharides: comparison with sulfated polysaccharides and other polyions." JOURNAL OF INFECTIOUS DISEASES. 164 (6), Dec. 1991, 1082-90.

17 I. Setnikar, et al., "Pharmacokinetics of glucosamine in the dog and in man." FOLIA ANGIOL. (25), 1977, 225-32.

18 I. Setnikar, et al., "Pharmacokinetics of glucosamine in man." ARZNEI-FORSCH. 43 (10), Oct. 1993, 1109-13.

19 Ibid.

20 G. Crystal, et al., "Stimulation of DNA synthesis by ascorbate in cultures of articular chondrocytes." ARTH. RHEUM. (25), 1982, 318-25.

21 I. Machtey and L. Ouaknine. "Tocopherol in osteoarthritis: a controlled pilot study." JOURNAL OF THE AMERICAN GERIATRICS SOCIETY. (26), 1978, 328-30.

22 Ibid. See also E. R. Schwartz, "The modulation of osteoarthritic development by vitamin C and E." INT. JOURNAL OF VIT. NUTR. RESEARCH. supplement, (26), 1984, 141-46.

23 R.R. Kulkani, et al., "Treatment of osteoarthritis with a herbomineral formulation: A double-blind, placebo-controlled, cross-over study." JOURNAL OF ETHNOPHARMACOLOGY. (33), 1991, 91-95. See also M.C.V. Lanhers et al., "Anti-inflammatory and analgesic effects of an aqueous extract of Harpagophytum procumbens. PLANTA MEDICA. (58), 1992, 117-23.

24 Rita Aquino, et al., "Plant metabolites, new compounds and anti-inflammatory activity of Uncaria tomentosa." JOURNAL OF NATURAL PRODUCTS. 54 (2), Mar-Apr. 1991, 453-59.

25 S.M. De Matta, et al., "Alkaloids and procyanidins of an Uncaria species from eastern Peru." FARMACO-SCI. 31 (7), July, 1976, 527-35.

26 James F. Balch. M.D. and Phyllis A. Balch, C.N.C. PRESCRIPTION FOR NUTRITIONAL HEALING. (Avery Publishing Group Inc., New York: 1990), 97.

27 G.B. Singh and C.K. Atal, "Pharmacology of an extract of salai guggal ex-Boswellia serrata, a new non-steroidal anti-inflammatory agent." AGENTS ACTION. (18), 1986, 407-12. See also C.K. Reddy, et al., "Studies on the metabolism of glycosaminoglycans under the influence of new herbal anti-inflammatory agents." BIOCHEMICAL PHARMACOLOGY. (20), 1989, 3527-34.

28 Kulkani, 91-95.

29 Michael T. Murray, THE HEALING POWER OF HERBS. (Prima Publishing, Rocklin, California: 1992-1995), 74.

30 Sid. Kircheimer. THE DOCTOR'S BOOK OF HOME REMEDIES. (Rodale Press, Emmaus, Pennsylvania: 1993), 228.

31 Gary Gagliardi, "Shark cartilage for achy joints." MUSCLE AND FITNESS. 56 (10), Oct. 1995, 52-57.

32 Dr. I. William Lane and Linda Comac. SHARKS DON'T GET CANCER. (Avery Publishing, Garden City, New York: 1993), 117-20.

33 R.L. Travers, et al., "Boron and arthritis: The results of a double-blind pilot study." JOURNAL NURT. MED. (1), 1990. 127-32.

34 R. Marcolongo, et al., "Double-blind multi center study of the activity of S-adenosyl-methionine in hip osteoarthritis." CURRENT THERAPEUTIC RESEARCH. (37), 1985, 82-94.

35 Michael Murray, N.D. and Joseph Pizzorno, N.D. ENCYCLOPEDIA OF NATURAL MEDICINE. (Prima Publishing, Rocklin, California: 1991), 450.

36 Ibid.